Herpes Simplex Virus

Managing HSV Holistically

RON KNESS

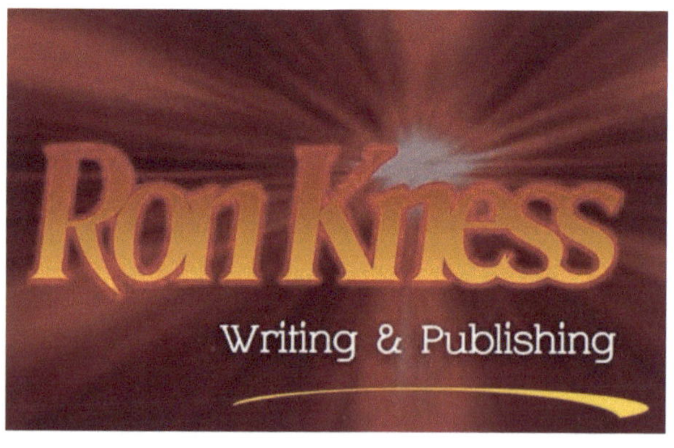

Contents

Disclaimer 1

Introduction..2

Just What is Herpes?..3

    Herpes and Pregnancy 9

Understanding How Herpes Is Transmitted 11

    Preventing the Spread 11

    Herpes and HIV 13

    Communication is Key...13

Medical Treatment for Herpes 17

Support Herpes Treatment Nutritionally 20

    Avoid Trigger Foods...21

    Add Support Foods 21

    Supplements to Consider...23

Minimize Herpes Outbreaks With Lifestyle and Natural Solutions 24

    Stress Management...24

    Chinese Medicine...25

    Essential Oils..26

Skincare 26

Sleep...27

Final Thoughts 28

Other Relevant Books by This Author 30

About the Author...36

Disclaimer

This publication is for informational purposes only and is not intended as medical advice. Medical advice should always be obtained from a qualified medical professional for any health conditions or symptoms associated with them.

Every possible effort has been made in preparing and researching this material. We make no warranties with respect to the accuracy, applicability of its contents or any omissions.

See your healthcare professional before starting any diet, health or exercise program!

Introduction

Herpes is a common sexually transmitted disease in the United States. In fact, one out of every six people ages 14 to 49 have this condition. But often people who suffer from herpes feel alone and ashamed.

Because herpes is a virus, it can be a lifelong battle with recurring outbreaks, embarrassment, and frustration. However, it doesn't have to be this way. There are many things you can do to combat herpes beyond prescription medication.

Using a holistic approach, you can work to manage your symptoms and prevent recurring outbreaks before they happen. This can reduce the overall stress and shame that you may have been carrying since your first outbreak.

In this book you'll learn more about herpes, what causes it and how it is transmitted. You'll also learn tips for prevention so that you can decrease the odds of becoming infected or infecting your partner if you already have it.

You'll find out more about herpes symptoms and how it is diagnosed. But most importantly, you'll discover a new way to approach and manage herpes beyond prescription medications.

With a combination of changes in nutrition, lifestyle, and proper use of prescription medications, you can have relief from herpes outbreaks and begin to feel healthier and more confident. We'll begin with the basics before we put it all together in the final chapter.

Just What is Herpes?

Herpes is a sexual transmitted disease (STD) that is caused by one of two viruses. The viruses are in the same family but are different in some important ways. They are called herpes simplex virus type 1 (HSV-1) and herpes simplex virus type 2 (HSV-2).

HSV-1 is actually the virus that causes oral herpes. That's the type that causes fever blisters and cold sores. A lot of people become infected with this during childhood or during their young adult years. However, through oral sex that type of virus can be transmitted to the genitals causing genital herpes symptoms.

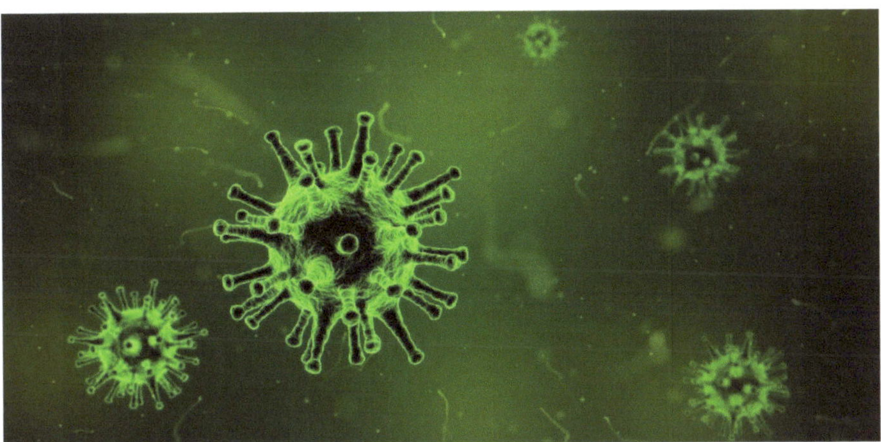

HSV-2 is the virus we associate with genital herpes. It is very contagious and can be spread by vaginal, anal, or oral sex. But it can also be transmitted through skin-on-skin contact with an open sore.

If you have HSV-1, it can be transmitted through saliva. HSV-2 is transmitted through genital secretions. Many people believe that you can only get herpes if your partner has a visible outbreak. However, you can get herpes even if your partner has no visible symptoms.

There are also many myths about herpes transmission that it's important to debunk. You cannot get herpes from swimming pools, toilet seats, bedding or towels. Contact must be more intimate than that.

Approximately 15% of people in the United States from ages 14 to 49 have been infected with HSV-2. It is more common in women with 1 in 5 women having it compared to 1 in 10 men. And lately it is also on the rise in the older populations like the baby boomers.

Many people who have the herpes virus have no symptoms. They may have no idea they even have herpes, so they are unaware that they are still able to transmit it to others. While you're more likely to transmit herpes during an outbreak, herpes can be transmitted even when you're asymptomatic.

Understanding Symptoms and Diagnosis

If you've possibly been exposed to herpes, you may be concerned about how to determine whether or not you have it. Knowing the symptoms can help. However, it's important to remember that many people have no symptoms even if they have contracted it.

If you experience an outbreak, the first one will usually be a few weeks after you were exposed and infected. The first outbreak is usually also the worst one that you'll have.

For women this can look like blisters and sores on the vagina, vulva, anus, buttocks, or thighs.

For men, the blisters may be seen on the penis, scrotum, anus, buttocks, or thighs. You may continue to get new sores for about a week after you see the first ones. And you can expect the symptoms to stick around for two or three weeks before subsiding.

In addition to blisters, there can be other symptoms. For example, you may experience pain when urinating and it may even at times seem difficult to urinate. Bowel movements may also be painful or uncomfortable.

Flu-like symptoms can also accompany an outbreak. You could have swollen lymph nodes especially in the groin area, joint pain, headaches, nausea, fever, and even vomiting.

Some people also describe having some mild symptoms before the blisters show up. They may feel tingling, itching, or pain in the buttocks, hips, or legs. The first outbreak tends to be the most severe and uncomfortable while future outbreaks are milder.

This virus stays in the body for life and unfortunately there is no cure for it. And it can continue to flare up over and over again if not treated right away. That's what makes it so important to look at holistic approaches so that you can have fewer and fewer outbreaks and control symptoms.

If you have symptoms, you definitely need to see your healthcare provider as soon as possible. They will be able to look at your symptoms and determine what tests need to be performed.

There are tests that can confirm if you have herpes or not. If you've been exposed to herpes, it is also a good idea to get tested for other sexually transmitted infections that can be passed along in the same way. In other words, the partner that gave you herpes could also be carrying other STDs too.

If you have a partner who has tested positive for herpes, but you have no symptoms, you should still play it safe and get tested to see if you have the infection also. If you do, you can discuss possible treatment options; if you don't have the infection, you can begin to take more steps to prevent getting it from your partner.

There are two tests that are used most commonly to diagnose herpes. The first is the PCR blood test. This test can tell you if you have herpes whether or not you are experiencing symptoms at the time of the test or not. It's a simple blood draw from the patient.

The blood is sent to the lab where it is tested for pieces of the herpes virus DNA. This test is considered very accurate and is the standard for diagnosing herpes.

If you have an outbreak with blisters and sores at the time, your doctor may perform a different test called a cell culture. With this test, the provider will take small sample of cells from an active sore and then that sample will be viewed under a microscope to look for the herpes simplex virus.

It is rare to have a false positive on these tests, but it can happen. If you have a low risk of getting herpes, you may want to request a second test. You can also have a false negative if you have been exposed to herpes recently enough that your body has not had a chance to for antibodies to develop in the bloodstream.

If you get a false negative, but you think you're at a high risk of having herpes transmission, it's a good idea to wait a few weeks and retest. In the meantime, you should act as if you have been infected when it comes to having protected sex. In the next chapter we'll discuss preventing transmission in more detail.

There are other tests that look for the virus in other body fluids such as saliva, urine, and tears. However, these tests are much more expensive to process and are used very rarely.

If you test positive for herpes, you might start to worry about the future of your health. For many people this can be embarrassing and there can be feelings of shame and guilt that go along with a positive diagnosis.

It's important to remember that herpes doesn't discriminate. It is simply a virus that has been passed from one person to another and this says nothing about who you are as a person. Sometimes these negative feelings can prevent individuals from seeking treatment.

It's essential that you work with your healthcare provider as soon as possible. There is much you can do to reduce symptoms, prevent future outbreaks, and prevent transmitting it to a current or future partner who isn't infected.

This diagnosis doesn't need to be the end of your good health or sex life. While there is no cure, there is treatment which can be highly effective.

Many people feel alone and isolated after a diagnosis. First, it's important to remember that herpes is a very common sexually transmitted disease. It's likely that you already know people who have it.

It's a good idea to reach out to family members or friends that you trust to discuss your diagnosis. You may also want to seek a support group where you can meet others who share your diagnosis and where you can ask questions and receive feedback as well as being able to lift up others.

There are even online support groups for people who have sexually transmitted diseases if you're interested in keeping things virtual. But in many large cities you can also find in-person groups.

The American Sexual Health Association provides an online listing of support groups in North America. You can access it here:
http://www.ashasexualhealth.org/stdsstis/herpes/support-groups/.

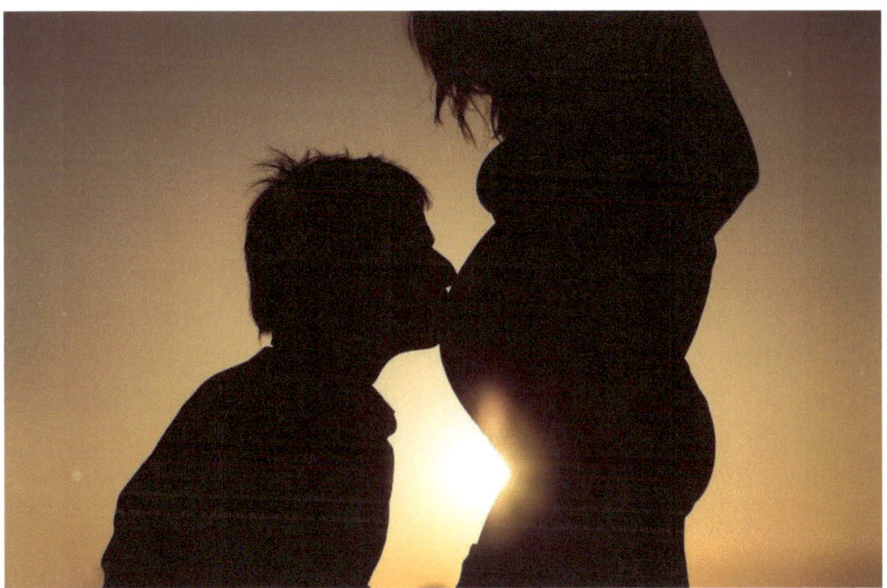

Herpes and Pregnancy

One special group that it's important to address is pregnant women. If you're pregnant and you think you may have herpes, it is critical that you talk with your doctor and get a true diagnosis.

In certain cases, genital herpes can cause some complications during pregnancy. Some research points to the idea that having genital herpes can lead to a miscarriage or early delivery. Additionally, herpes can be passed to your baby.

While it's possible for your baby to become exposed to herpes during pregnancy, it's more likely that it can happen during childbirth. As the baby passes through the birth canal, it can come in contact with the tissues that transmit genital herpes.

If the baby is infected at birth, there can be serious, even deadly consequences. When babies develop herpes, it is called neonatal herpes. Babies who are exposed must be treated right away and even if they are treated, there can be long-term complications and even death.

The good news is that babies can avoid this exposure by being delivered via C-section. This allows the baby to be born without exposure to the virus. Women who are treated with antiviral mediations also have fewer problems with outbreaks and possibly avoid a C-section delivery.

Understanding How Herpes Is Transmitted

Herpes is a virus that can be transmitted from skin-to-skin and through sexual contact. The only way to guarantee that you don't become infected with it or transmit your infection to someone else is to avoid all sexual contact.

However in reality, most people will have sex because for most of us having an active sex life is part of our overall wellness. But to prevent transmission, you'll want to practice using protection during all sexual activity.

Preventing the Spread

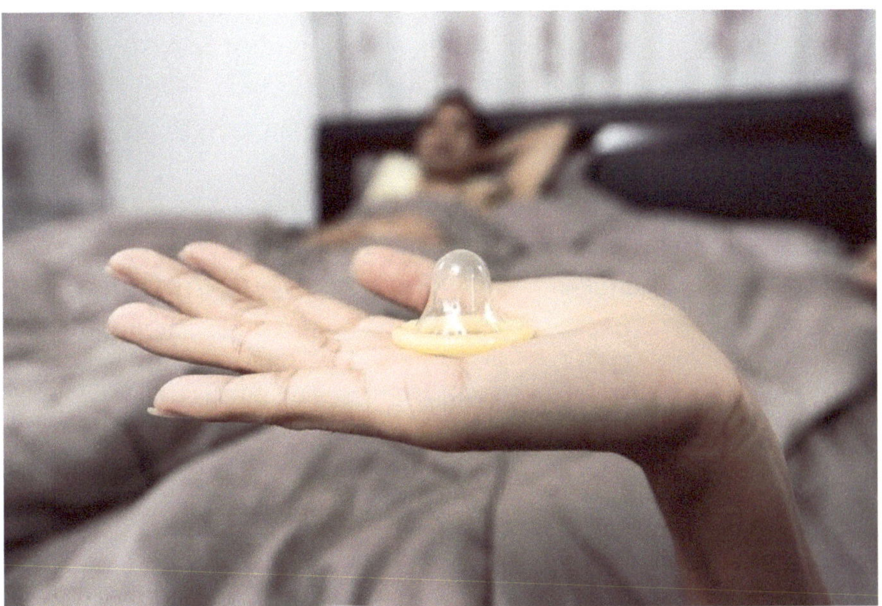

As mentioned before, herpes can be spread through oral, anal, or vaginal sex. It's important to use condoms correctly and use them every time you have sex with a partner. Additionally, you'll need to use dental dams when participating in oral sex.

Condoms won't always protect you because herpes can live on parts of the body that condoms don't cover. For example, the scrotum, thighs, labia, and buttocks can all carry herpes virus. But using condoms will significantly decrease your risk of transmission.

If you or your partner has a herpes outbreak, you should not have sex during the outbreak. This is when herpes transmission is most likely to occur. Even using a condom will not be protective enough at this time.

As the outbreak begins to calm down and go away, wait to have sex until all sores are completely gone and healed. Scabs should also have all fallen off. You should also avoid touching the herpes sores on your own body because you can spread the infection to other parts of your body this way.

During an outbreak, handwashing is critical after touching any area that is infected. It's important to use soap and water and wash for at least 20 seconds to insure you don't pass the virus on to other parts of your body or to a partner.

If you or your partner have herpes, it's important to pay attention to signs that an outbreak is about to occur. Burning, itching, and tingling can often occur before the sores actually show up. During this time, you should stop having sex and then wait until the outbreak has completely healed before resuming sexual activity.

When it comes to HSV-1, it's important to avoid kissing anyone when you have a cold sore on your mouth or if you feel one coming on. Additionally, if you wear contact lenses avoid any temptation to use saliva to wet them. This can spread herpes infection to your eye.

Even when you're feeling well, and you don't see any signs of an outbreak, it's important to practice protected sex with condoms and dental dams every time so that you reduce your risk of transmission.

Herpes and HIV

It's important to discuss HIV prevention while on the subject of herpes. According to Planned Parenthood, people who have herpes are twice as likely to get HIV as people who do not have the virus.

And if a person has herpes and HIV, there is a greater likelihood of passing the herpes on to sexual partners. This makes it critical to use condoms correctly and consistently to protect yourself and your partner from possible infection of either disease.
(https://www.plannedparenthood.org/learn/stds-hiv-safer-sex/herpes/how-is-herpes-prevented)

Communication is Key

So far, we've discussed the mechanics of how the virus is transmitted and how you can prevent it. But none of that information does any good if you don't communicate with your partner.

Telling a partner you have herpes can be challenging and a difficult conversation to have. You may also fear asking your partner about their own disease status. But having these conversations can be the key to good health and the prevention of herpes as well as other sexually transmitted diseases.

You may worry that your days of romance are over and that this disease will put an end to your sex life, but that doesn't have to be true. Being able to discuss your sexual health is an important step toward better intimacy with a partner.

You may want to start by asking your partner if they have ever been tested for sexually transmitted infections. Then it's easier to discuss that you've been tested and actually do have a chronic issue.

When you're ready to discuss herpes, it can also help to have educational brochures so your partner doesn't just have to take your word for it. Also make sure you share that you want to be up front about this so that you protect your partner.

Timing is also crucial when it comes to having this conversation. This should be a private conversation that happens without interruptions. It should also happen before you've done anything that puts your partner at risk if possible. If you've already had a sexual relationship and then were diagnosed later, this isn't something you can do. But if you haven't embarked on a sexual relationship yet, it's important to discuss this first.

You don't need to tell someone the first time you meet that you have herpes. But you do owe your partner honesty if your relationship is on the road to becoming intimate.

While you can't control your partner's reaction, you can feel good about being honest. It's possible your partner will be understanding and happy to work with you to have protected sex and allow your relationship to develop.

But it's also possible that your partner will react negatively and decide this relationship isn't for them. If that happens it can be very heartbreaking, but it's better to have this happen as early in the relationship as possible rather than later when the relationship is more fully developed.

Remember, too, that some people need time to process this kind of new information. You may have a partner who freaks out right when you tell them the news, but after having some time to process and reflect will be okay with it later.

If you're already having sex and you find out that you have herpes, it's important to have this conversation and that both of you get tested. It's hard to say when someone actually contracts herpes because it can live in the body for weeks, months, or even years without an outbreak.

Avoid the temptation to try and blame someone for giving you herpes or accusing them of cheating. That is in the past and there is nothing you can do about it now. Instead, focus on dealing with the reality at hand, on getting a proper diagnosis and starting appropriate treatment.

When you're diagnosed with herpes, it's also important to talk to your previous sexual partners so that they know they need to get tested as well. It would be best to talk to each person directly and as soon as possible.

But if you don't feel you can do that, one option is to talk to your local health department about possible partner notification services. Additionally, you can use online partner notification services that are anonymous. While it is not as good as having that conversation face-to-face, it is better than no notification at all.

It would be better to get some kind of notification rather than none, but getting an anonymous text or email about an STD can be pretty shocking. If at all possible, muster up the courage and make the notification personally.

One final note about safety. If you think your partner or a previous partner might become violent upon hearing this news, it's best to protect your own safety first. This would be the one case where an anonymous service might be the best choice.

Medical Treatment for Herpes

Once you've been diagnosed with herpes, it's important to first seek medical treatment. Many clinics that perform herpes testing also provide treatment. While there is no cure, the medical system does offer some assistance. In later chapters we'll discuss more holistic approaches as well.

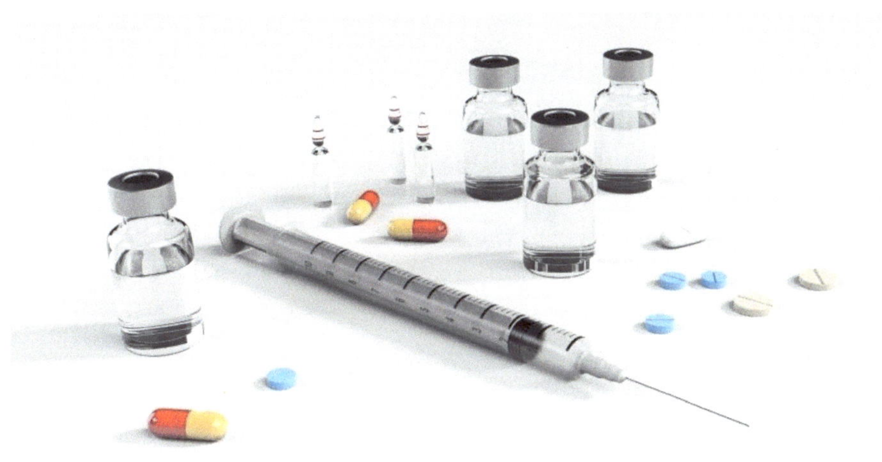

The drugs most commonly used to treat herpes are antiviral medications that work to keep viruses from reproducing. If they can't reproduce, they can't harm your body. The most common drugs are acyclovir known by the brand name Zovirax, valcacyclovir known by the brand name Vatrex, and famciclovir know by the brand name Famvir.

All three of these medications are given in pill form. However, in some extreme cases acyclovir can be given intravenously. In most cases you'll be given the option of using pills.

There are different types of medical treatment depending on where you are in the disease process. When you're first diagnosed and are symptomatic, you'll be given antiviral medications. This first course will last anywhere from seven to 10 days.

This first course will help to stop the outbreak and give you relief from the sores. If you still have sores at the end of the medication course, your doctor may prescribe more until all of the sores are gone and completely healed.

After you have the initial outbreak under control, you have a couple of choices about how to proceed. Your doctor may prescribe antiviral medications that you can keep in your medicine cabinet until you have an outbreak.

This type of treatment is called intermittent therapy. You'll begin medication as soon as you see signs of an outbreak coming on. You'll still probably have sores, however, using the medication can shorten the time of your outbreak and make it less severe.

The other type of treatment is known as suppressive treatment. This is an option if you're experiencing a lot of outbreaks. With this type of therapy, you'll take an antiviral medication daily. This can reduce the overall number of outbreaks and for some people this keeps them completely at bay.

Most doctors won't prescribe suppressive treatment unless you have at least six outbreaks in a single calendar year. However, if you have fewer, but they're severe, your doctor may go ahead and consider this form of treatment.

The main thing to know about medical treatment is that there isn't a one size fits all approach. You'll need to work with your healthcare provider to determine which one is best for you.

One issue with medication is that it always comes with some side effects. These antiviral drugs typically have mild side effects and research supports using them for long periods of time.

The most common symptoms include headaches, dizziness, fatigue, and nausea. If you struggle with severe side effects, you should talk with your healthcare provider about changing the regimen.

Finally, you can reduce your dependence on medications by making some nutritional and lifestyle changes that support a healthy immune system. A holistic approach will give you the best possible outcome.

Support Herpes Treatment Nutritionally

It might seem strange to think about, but nutrition really can make a big impact on the status of your herpes disease. There are many ways you can improve your diet to keep outbreaks at bay.

When it comes to nutrition, there are several goals. Proper nutrition can help to literally stop the virus. But it can also work to improve the health of your skin and your immune system so that the herpes virus has a harder time taking over. Good nutrition can also eliminate triggers that lead to outbreaks.

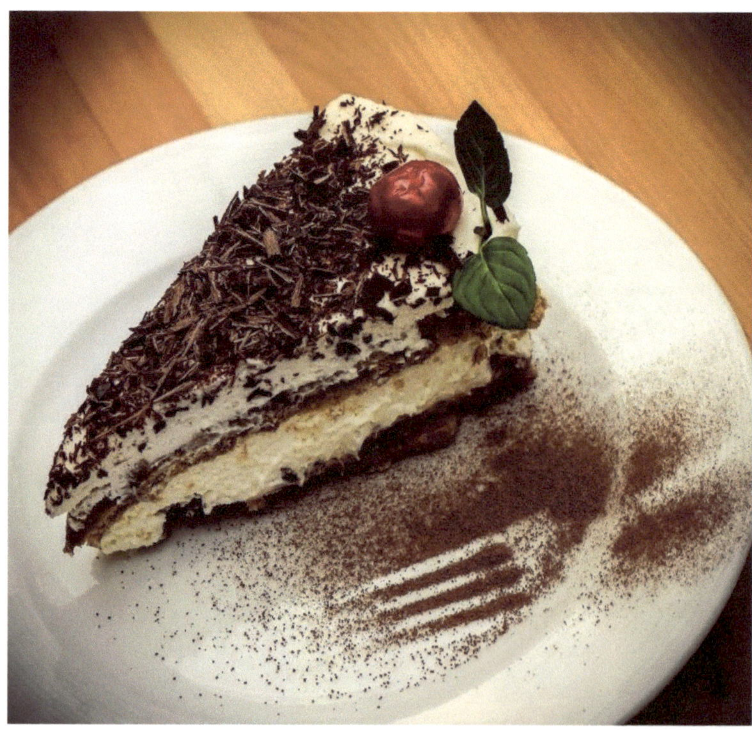

Avoid Trigger Foods

Some foods are known to trigger herpes for many people. One chemical to avoid is arginine which is a natural amino acid. It can be found in chocolate, nuts, oats, and protein supplements that contain it. This amino acid helps the herpes simplex grow and can lead to an outbreak.

Artificial sweeteners can also be problematic. A few other foods to avoid include white bread, refined sugars, coffee, caffeine, and sodas. Alcohol should be used in moderation.

You may also find it helpful to keep a [food diary](https://journalingforfun.com/product/52-week-journal-for-health-and-fitness/) and when you have an outbreak look at the foods you were eating at that time. It's probably not one food that leads to the outbreak but rather a pattern of eating. This information can help you to determine individually what you need to avoid.

Add Support Foods

While there are some foods to avoid as mentioned above, you'll find more success in focusing on adding foods that are supportive of your health. For example, eating foods that contain high amounts of lysine can be very beneficial.

Lysine is an amino acid that actually stops the herpes simplex virus from reproducing. By adding this you can reduce the number of outbreaks you have as well as decrease their intensity.

You can take a lysine supplement, but you can also find it in food such as most vegetables, dairy products, eggs, brewer's yeast, sardines, cod, chicken, beef, lamb, and sprouts.

Beets, mangoes, apples, apricots, avocados, and figs are particularly high.

It's also helpful to eat foods that support good skin health. This includes zinc, bioflavonoids, and vitamin C. Some foods to add include citrus fruits, broccoli, Brussels sprouts, strawberries, beans, lentils, black tea, grape juice, and pumpkin seeds.

Eating foods that are high in nutrients, especially vitamins, will support a strong immune system (*https://www.amazon.com/Power-Your-Immune-System-Year-round/dp/1534842349*). Fresh juices (*https://www.amazon.com/Juicing-Your-Way-Better-Health/dp/1537550993*), vegetables, especially leafy vegetables, and raw fruits can all be beneficial. Aim to eat a colorful diet filled with a wide variety of vitamins and antioxidants.

Water is also critical for good health. You need to drink adequate water to flush out toxins and help your cells perform optimally. However, you also need to drink water that is alkaline and that is filtered properly.

Look for water that is filtered but still contains minerals. Also consider adding lemon juice or lime juice (*https://www.amazon.com/Make-Your-Own-Infused-Water-ebook/dp/B074D4WL2T*) to help alkalinize the body. This makes it more difficult for the virus to take hold.

Supplements to Consider

While it's usually best to get nutrition from actual food, there are some supplements you might want to consider. L-lysine can be taken daily to help reduce oral herpes symptoms and outbreaks. Monolaurin is a supplement that is also antiviral.

Vitamin C supports good immune system functioning as well as healthy skin. Zinc can be taken as a supplement to boost your immunity as well. Stress is a known trigger for herpes and taking a B-complex vitamin can protect you from the effects of stress.

You may also want to consider herbs that have antiviral properties such as garlic, Echinacea, elderberry, and licorice root. It's always a good idea to speak with a healthcare provider before beginning any supplements to make sure they don't counteract any medications or health conditions you currently experience.

Minimize Herpes Outbreaks With Lifestyle and Natural Solutions

In addition to eating a healthy diet and supporting your body with good nutrition, there are other lifestyle factors that can improve your health and help prevent outbreaks. In this chapter we'll look at a variety of ways you can make small changes that have a big impact on your health.

Stress Management

Stress is one of the top contributors to suppressing the immune system and opening yourself up for a herpes outbreak. It's critical to remove as many stressors from your life as possible and practice good stress management (*https://www.amazon.com/Stress-Your-Health-Recognize-Symptoms/dp/1539766071*) techniques.

Exercise, spending time with friends, relaxing with a good book, and generally taking part in hobbies that you enjoy can all help you to experience stress relief. You may also find that counseling with a good therapist will help you to manage emotions.

You may also consider adding yoga or some sort of meditation or mindfulness (*https://www.amazon.com/Power-Mindfulness-Control-Your-Conrol/dp/1539575543*) practice to your daily routine. This can help you to release tension and relax your mind and body. Guided imagery and hypnosis may also be beneficial.

Having herpes alone can add stress to your life. Getting some help to work through your emotions is helpful. Herpes is simply an illness caused by a virus but there can be shame and stigma attached to it.

Those feelings can exacerbate your stress and lead to more outbreaks which in turn cause more stress and lead to more outbreaks. Stopping this vicious cycle is imperative to maintain long term good health.

Chinese Medicine

Chinese medicine is a wonderful way to balance the body and shore up your immune system. When you see a Chinese medicine practitioner you may be prescribed herbs, acupuncture, cupping, and other ways to clear your energy.

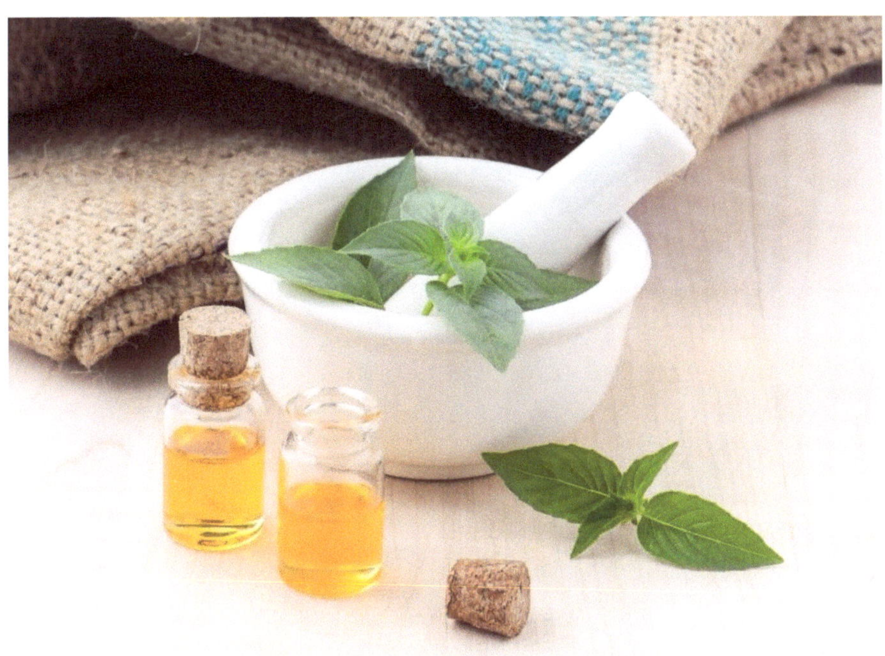

Essential Oils

[Essential oils](https://www.amazon.com/Essential-Oils-Health-Healing-Conditions/dp/1542359007) (*https://www.amazon.com/Essential-Oils-Health-Healing-Conditions/dp/1542359007*) have become very popular as natural medicine. When it comes to herpes there are essential oils that can both treat herpes and boost the immune system in general.

Clove, myrrh, and tea tree oil are all antiviral and can be applied to sores. Small amounts can be applied directly but if you find them to be painful, you can dilute the essential oils with coconut or grapeseed oil.

Diffusing essential oils provides aromatherapy that can boost your immune system. Tea tree oil, eucalyptus globulus, frankincense, scots pine, and rosemary are all appropriate to diffuse for this purpose.

Skincare

Quality skincare can help keep your skin strong when you don't have an outbreak, but it can also help outbreaks heal faster and have less pain. You should use natural, mild soap such as castile soap to wash and use warm water to rinse.

Sitting in a warm bath or taking a shower can provide heat that decreases the pain. You can also warm a towel fresh from the dryer and press it to the affected area to give some relief. During an outbreak, wear comfortable clothes that are loose so that your sores don't experience friction and they can get air.

When it comes to drying after a bath or shower, use one towel for any areas that are covered in blisters and sores. Then use another for areas that haven't been affected. This prevents the spread of the virus to new areas.

Sleep

Getting consistent quality sleep (*https://www.amazon.com/Clean-Sleeping-Health-Affect-Appearance/dp/1542481031*) of at least 7-9 hours each night gives your body the time it needs to repair and restore at the cellular level. This will support your body in fighting the herpes virus.

Final Thoughts

Being diagnosed with herpes or having a partner diagnosed can be shocking. You may feel initially your world has been turned upside down. But herpes isn't a death sentence ... though it can be a chronic condition.

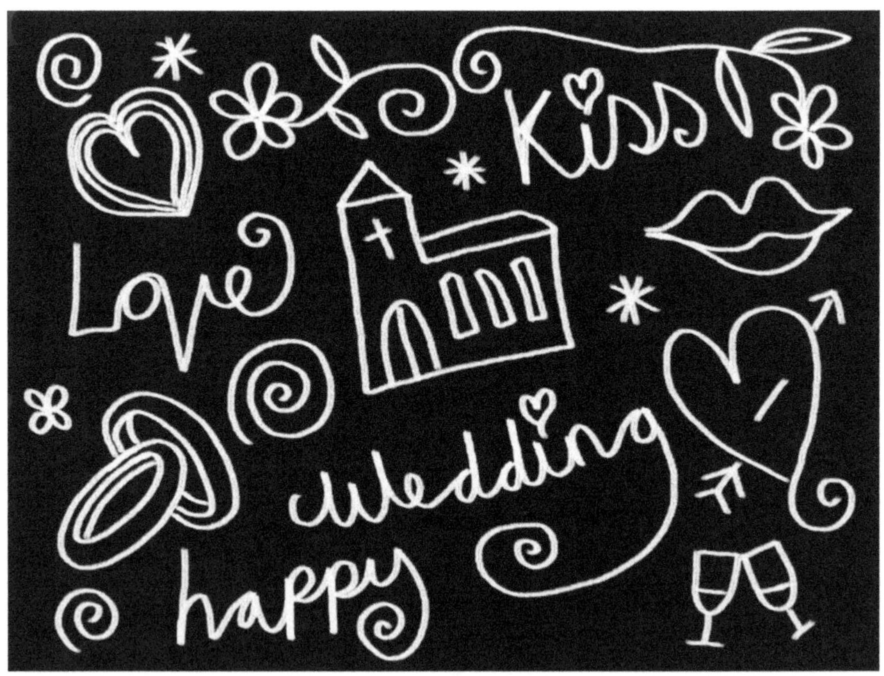

Give yourself some time to process the news and then learn all you can about it. In this book you've learned the basics of what herpes is, how it's transmitted, and how it can be treated.

Now it's your turn to choose what methods you'll use for preventing the transmission of herpes to someone else, or possibly you, if a partner has herpes.

You also must decide how you'll communicate about this disease and make sure that your emotional needs are met.

If you have herpes you'll also want to do your best to develop a strong, healthy immune system so that you can reduce the number of outbreaks you experience and also keep outbreaks as mild as possible.

You can make the illness much more uncomfortable by living a low stress lifestyle. If you work on staying in the moment and taking care of your body overall, you can minimize your discomfort and even get to the point that herpes isn't at the forefront of your mind.

Herpes is nothing that you would ever wish to have or hope to have, but if you do have to face it, know that you are not alone. Don't be afraid to reach out and seek support. Reach out to family and friends you trust and look for support from groups designed to help you during this time.

When you take care of your mental health, your physical health will respond well. Herpes isn't a moral issue or one that should make you feel ashamed. But by acknowledging negative feelings and working through them you can let go of them and build upon a more positive foundation.

When you're initially diagnosed with herpes it can be all consuming. But it doesn't have to stay that way. In the beginning, though, you will need to take time to learn more about your illness and make some changes.

By taking the time to make some lifestyle changes and work on your own health, you'll eventually get to a new normal. And that new normal will include happiness, joy, fulfillment, fun, and good health.

Other Relevant Books by This Author

If you would like to read more relevant books about this topic, here is a list of the CreateSpace links, titles and descriptions from this author:

https://www.amazon.com/Lyme-Disease-Symptoms-Treatment-Mis-Diagnosed/dp/1545339937

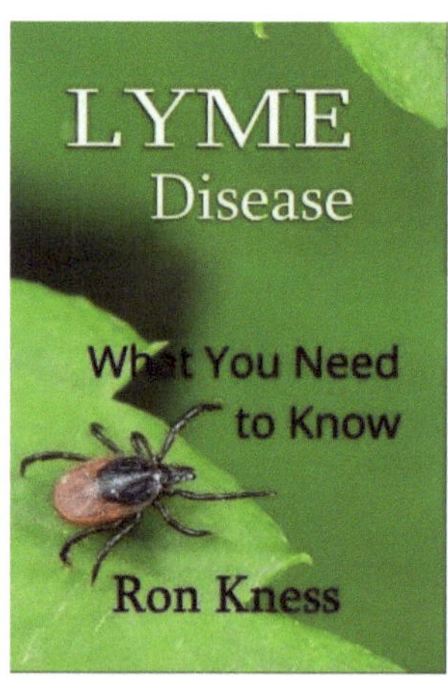

Lyme Disease - What You Need to Know: Cause, Symptoms and Treatment for This Often Mis-Diagnosed Disease

We want to be more empowered concerning our health. We also want to be more educated about Lyme Disease. And we want to prevent, recognize the symptoms and know how to treat Lyme Disease!

We can achieve ALL of these goals with the newest release from Ron Kness called "Lyme Disease - What You Need To Know".

Based on these exciting teachings, you will learn about all the dramatic benefits of preventing getting it in the first place, however, recognizing the signs of it if you happen to get it.

This book is built around a very clear, concept: what you need to know about Lyme Disease. It's not just about recognizing the signs of Lyme Disease. It is also about taking precautions in the first place. I

n this book, we look at all of the ways you can protect your health by taking precautions when in tick habitat, starting with recognizing ticks that carry the disease. This book will also look at the many other steps that can be taken to support this goal, from reading this book to adhering to the advice in it. Treating Lyme Disease early has a greater positive impact on your health rather than later after it has become Chronic Lyme Disease.

In "Lyme Disease - What You Need To Know", we'll cover all the bases, giving you everything you need to know to recognize the symptoms of Lyme Disease.

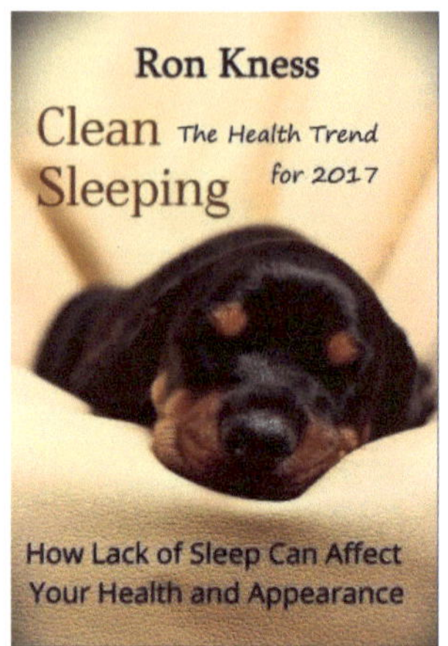

Clean Sleeping - The Health Trend for 2017: How Lack of Sleep Can Affect Your Health and Appearance

We want to be more energetic the next day . We also want to be more productive . And we want to get more sleep and of a better quality! We can achieve ALL of these goals with the newest release from Ron Kness called Clean Sleeping - The Health Trend For 2017.

Based on these exciting teachings, you will learn about all the dramatic benefits of restful sleep and eating foods that help people sleep better. This book is built around a very clear, concept: feel well rested. It's not just about ways to get the maximum amount of restorative sleep.

Having great sleeping habits is linked to eating healthy. This is because some foods are more conducive to sleeping well than others In this book, we look at all of the ways you can improve your own sleeping habits, starting with calming the mind.

This book will also look at the many other steps that can be taken to support this goal, from doing meditation before retiring for the night to taking a warm bath scented with an essential oil and listening to soft music.

Even the choices you make about healthy eating and creating sleep-inducing bedroom environment can have an impact on your sleeping habits. In Clean Sleeping - The Health Trend For 2017, we'll cover all the bases, giving you everything you need to know to get the maximum amount of quality sleep each night.

It is the most important thing you can do for your overall physical and mental health. The good news is that getting a good night's rest is totally doable ... we show you how!

https://www.amazon.com/Mindful-Eating-Mindfully-Emotional-Physical/dp/1975988930

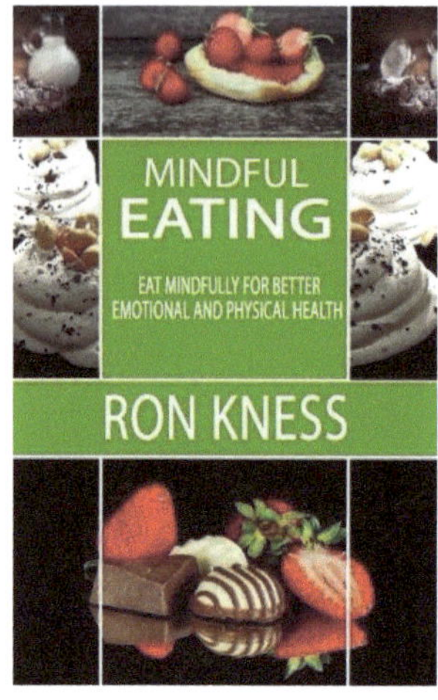

Mindful Eating: Eat Mindfully for Better Emotional and Physical Health

This book could be your key to better health! What type of person are you when it comes to eating? There's two main types of eaters in this world, there's the type who are conscious of every bite they put in their mouth … and then there's the people who eat without realizing what or how much they are eating. Which type of person are you?

If you are the latter type, this book is for you. It's 100% your choice. But frankly, if you're struggling with your emotional health, physical health, or both - learning how to eat mindfully could help improve it. If all of your efforts to resolve your health problems have not yielded the results you have been looking for, what do you have to lose!

In this book, we … - Define Mindful (and Mindless) Eating - Talk About Why Junk and Processed Food Is So Addictive - Discuss the 6 Pillars of Mindful Eating - Gain an Understanding the 7 Different Types of Hunger - Discover How Much Food You Really Need - Deal with Withdrawal, Cravings and Slip-Ups - Learn How to Live and Move Mindfully to Complement Our Your New Eating Program

And the ***Mindful Eating Guide*** is complemented by 5 other free downloads, making it a complete eating program ... - Junk Food Alternatives - Healthy Foods List - Mindful Questions to Ask Yourself Before Eating - Training Your Brain - Mindful Eating Checklist. Get your copy today!

About the Author

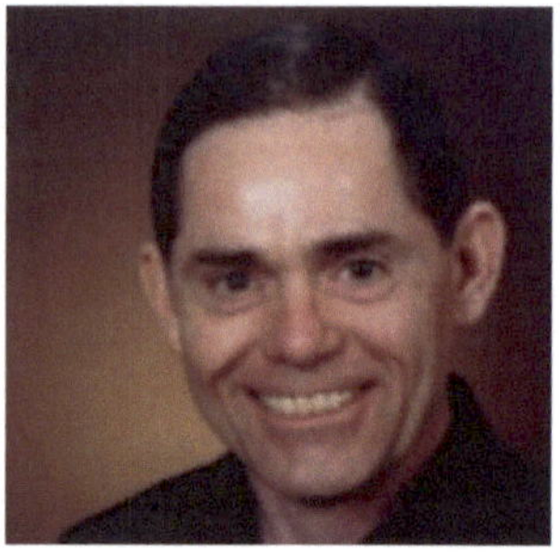

I have published books on Amazon for Kindle, CreateSpace and various other publishing platforms.

While most of my books are on health and fitness in general, as I age (now mid-60s at the time of this writing) my topics of interest are geared toward aging baby boomers and older.

Besides my own writing, I also ghostwrite ebooks, books, reports, articles, blogs and do Kindle conversions for clients on a variety of topics.

Today my wife and I are retired from our careers and live in Gold Canyon, AZ. I now write as a retirement business where you'll find me happily sitting in my office typing away on my laptop as I work on my next book or ghostwriting project . . . that is if we are not traveling on a cruise ship - our new-found mode of travel.